Reverse Lymphedema Now

The 5 Essentials for Self-Care at Home

"Take control of lymphedema at home!"

By Mateo Estevez PT, CLT

Copyright © 2023 by Mateo Estevez CLT, PT

All rights reserved.

No part of this book may be reproduced, stored in a retrieval system, or transmitted in any form or by any means, electronic, mechanical, photocopying, recording, or otherwise, without the prior written permission of the publisher.

Why was this book written?

Lymphedema affects over 250 million people worldwide, making it a genuine global health concern. Even though treating lymphatic problems is incredibly expensive for the healthcare system, very few doctors have the necessary training. Three to five million Americans will have lymphedema by the year 2022. Of the estimated 5 million Americans who have lymphedema, it is unknown how many do not have health insurance. However, we can assume that 1 in 100,000 persons worldwide and 1 in 1000 Americans suffer from lymphedema. This book was written for these people!

It didn't take a statistician to see that there was a need for those who didn't have insurance or didn't have access to qualified care for lymphedema management. As I continued to work in the field as a lymphedema expert, I saw that many of the patients I was directed to had never seen a lymphedema specialist despite having lymphedema for years. This was the tipping point that prompted me to create this book. Later, I discovered that the lymphatic system is only briefly covered in medical school. Many doctors simply do not receive the training required to properly identify and treat lymphedema. This book aims to fill the gap in providing expert guidance for persons suffering from lymphedema.

The purpose of this book

The purpose of this book is to explain the essentials of treating lymphedema safely and successfully at home. It also intends to teach you how to treat your lymphedema by providing accessible and straightforward guidelines. Remember, if possible, speak with a qualified lymphedema physical therapist or a doctor in your area.

About the author

I am a certified lymphedema physical therapy specialist with more than 20 years of combined lymphedema and rehabilitation experience. Specifically, I have many years of experience treating lymphedema in the home. I currently run a small lymphedema home health business in Orlando, Florida. My passion is helping those who suffer from lymphedema.

You can reach me at mestevez@flo-motionlymphedema.com

Book Format

Throughout this book, you will find helpful tables and illustrations to serve as quick learning tools and summarize the most important aspects of self-care. In this book, you will find some open space for you to take notes, comments, or write questions to discuss with your healthcare provider. The book is designed to be a learning experience. I encourage you to be as interactive as possible.

Good Luck, and God Bless!

Follow us on social media:
Facebook: Flo-Motion Lymphedema Home Therapy Specialists
Instagram: flo_motion_lymphedema_therapy

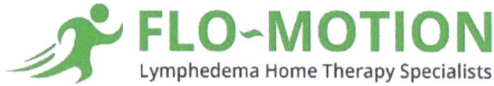

List of Tables:

Table 1 | The stages of lymphedema and their differences 12
Table 2 | The 5 essentials of treating lymphedema at home 14
Table 3 | Compression options for self-care at home 23
Table 4 | The most common processed foods 26
Table 5 | Strategies for water intake at home 28
Table 6 | Example of an ultra-low sodium 7-day meal plan used during flare-ups 29
Table 7 | Example of a low sodium 7-day meal plan that can be maintained all year around ... 30
Table 8 | Low-pH lotions 32
Table 9 | Assistive skin care and dressing tools for self-care at home 33
Table 10 | Fundamental home exercises for lymphedema self-care at home 35
Table 11 | Essentials for traveling with lymphedema 44
Table 12 | Lymphedema emergency supply kit 47

List of Figures:

Figure 1 | The lymphatic system - note the high concentrations of lymph nodes in the neck, armpit, and groin - NAG for short 9
Figure 2 | The lymph nodes help to move and filter fluid 9
Figure 3 | A positive stemmer's sign on the right lower extremity and a negative on the left .. 11
Figure 4 | The first 3 three stages of lymphedema are reversible with early intervention 12
Figure 5 | The lymphatic fluid pathways called watersheds 17
Figure 6 | Node clearing of the neck, armpit, and groin (NAG) 19
Figure 7 | Diaphragmatic/belly breathing improves the lymphatic flow of the trunk 20
Figure 8 | When fluids are compressed, the flow rate increases 22
Figure 9 | Adjustable Velcro garments - the best option for flare-ups and daily care at home. 23
Figure 10 | There are several strategies for water intake at home 28
Figure 11 | Home Exercise Program (HEP) for daily maintenance of lymphedema 36
Figure 12 | Walking creates a calf muscle pump for lower extremity lymphatic flow 40
Figure 13 | Elevation is an essential part of lymphedema self-care at home 42
Figure 14 | Pneumatic compression pumps - an effective way to safely manage lymphedema 46
Figure 15 | Cellulitis is caused by even a minor breach in skin integrity 52

Table of Contents

Chapter 1: Lymphedema Introduction 8
- Causes of Lymphedema 8
- Symptoms of Lymphedema 10
- Treatment of Lymphedema 10
- Diagnosis of Lymphedema 11
- Stages of Lymphedema 11

Chapter 2: Lymphedema Self-Care Overview 15
- The Importance of Healthy Weight? 15
- Keeping the Skin Safe 15
- Avoid Wearing Restricted Clothes 16
- The Use of Good Hygiene 16
- Exercise Frequently 16

Chapter 3: Manual Lymphatic Drainage Therapy 17
- How Does Manual Lymphatic Drainage Therapy Work? 17
- How Effective is MLD Therapy? 18
- MLD Therapy is Beneficial for Whom? 18
- Node Clearing Exercises 19
- Diaphragmatic Breathing 19

Chapter 4: Compression Garments 21
- What Exactly are Compression Garments? 21
- How Does Compression Function? 21
- Selecting the Best Compression Garments 22
- Maintaining Compression Garments 24

Chapter 5: Nutrition and Lymphedema 25
- The Role of Nutrition in Lymphedema Management 25
- Lifestyle Variables Affecting Lymphedema Symptoms 27
- The Importance of Hydration and Lymphedema 27

Chapter 6: Skin Care and Lymphedema 31
- Skin Examinations Every Day 31
- Suitable Skin Washing 31
- Application of Low-pH Moisturizer 31

Chapter 7: Exercise and Lymphedema 34

 Advantages of Exercise 34

 Safety Measures for Exercise 34

 Tips for Exercise for Lymphedema 34

Chapter 8: Elevation 41

 What Happens During Elevation? 41

Chapter 9: Traveling with Lymphedema 43

 Tips for Comfortable and Safe Travel 43

 Travel Safety Precautions and Precautions to Take 43

 How to be Ready for Unexpected Situations While Traveling 43

Chapter 10: Preventing and Managing Lymphedema Re-congestion or Flare-Ups 45

 Lymphedema Triggers 45

 How to Prevent Re-congestion or Flare-ups 45

 What to Do Right Away When Lymphedema Flares-up 46

 Making a Lymphedema First Aid Emergency Kit 47

Chapter 11: Dealing with Minor Skin Breaks and Tears at Home 49

 Preventing Skin Breaks and Early Detection 49

 How to Clean and Bandage Minor Skin Breaks 49

 Compression During the Healing Process 49

 Preventing Another Skin Break 50

Chapter 12: Common Lymphedema Complications 51

 Cellulitis 51

 Lymphangitis 52

Chapter 13. The Emotional & Mental Impact of Lymphedema 54

 The Effects of Lymphedema on the Psyche 54

 Techniques for Managing Emotional & Mental Impact of Lymphedema 55

Chapter 14: Living with Lymphedema 57

Chapter 15: Lymphedema Management in the Future 59

 Research Advances in Lymphedema 59

 Innovations in the Management of Lymphedema 59

Chapter 16: Final Reflections 61

Resources 64

Chapter 1: Lymphedema Introduction

Lymphedema is a condition that affects millions of people around the world. It develops when the lymphatic system, responsible for draining fluid from tissues, becomes damaged or compromised. The result is a buildup of lymphatic fluid in the affected area, causing swelling, discomfort, and other symptoms.

Causes of Lymphedema

Lymphedema can have several underlying causes, including:

1. Surgery: Lymphedema can occur because of surgical procedures that involve the removal of lymph nodes, such as breast cancer surgery or melanoma surgery.

2. Radiation therapy: Radiation can damage the lymphatic system, leading to lymphedema.

3. Infection: Inflammatory responses to infections can damage the lymphatic vessels, such as cellulitis

4. Inherited conditions: Some individuals may be predisposed to lymphedema due to a genetic disorder that affects their lymphatic system, such as primary lymphedema.

5. Morbid Obesity: Being severely overweight can damage the lymphatic system.

Let's get an essential understanding of lymphatic anatomy. The following figures give an overview of the lymphatic system as it pertains to self-care at home. It's important to understand the location of the lymph nodes, and that stimulating them helps to move fluid.

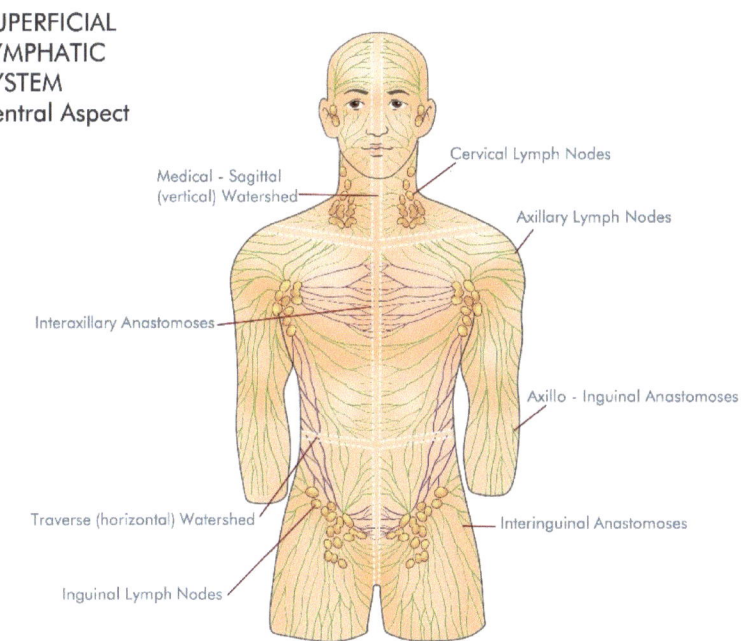

Figure 1 | The lymphatic system - note the high concentrations of lymph nodes in the neck, armpit, and groin - NAG for short

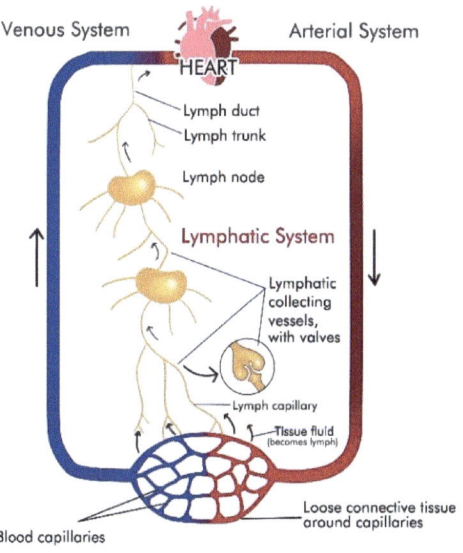

Figure 2 | The lymph nodes help to move and filter fluid

Symptoms of Lymphedema

Lymphedema symptoms vary in severity depending on the affected area. Some common symptoms include:

1. Swelling in the affected area, such as the arm or leg with one side more pronounced
2. Heaviness or tightness in the affected area
3. Limited range of motion in the affected area
4. Aching or discomfort in the affected area
5. Skin changes, such as thickening or hardening of the skin
6. Recurrent infections in the affected area

Treatment of Lymphedema

There is currently no cure for lymphedema, but a range of treatment options can help manage symptoms and improve quality of life. Commonly used treatment options include:

1. **Compression therapy**: Compression garments or bandages can reduce swelling and improve lymphatic function. a. Adjustable Velcro garments b. Compression socks
2. **Manual lymphatic drainage**: A specialized massage technique that can help move lymphatic fluid out of the affected area. There are great videos available on this subject on YouTube. Just make sure the content creator is a CLT (Certified Lymphedema Therapist)
    - Node clearing
    - Self-massage
3. **Exercise**: Gentle active range of motion exercise, such as walking or swimming, can improve lymphatic function and reduce swelling.
4. **Surgery**: In severe cases of lymphedema, surgical removal of excess tissue can improve lymphatic flow.

Diagnosis of Lymphedema

With a nearly 90% accuracy rate, the Stemmer's sign is an excellent way to tell if someone has lymphedema. It is almost impossible to have a false positive Stemmer's sign due to the effect of protein-rich lymph fluid on the skin's elasticity on the top of the foot, toes, or middle finger. Over time, static lymph fluid accumulation under the skin can cause hardening, density, and fibrosis of the skin, making it impossible to pinch.

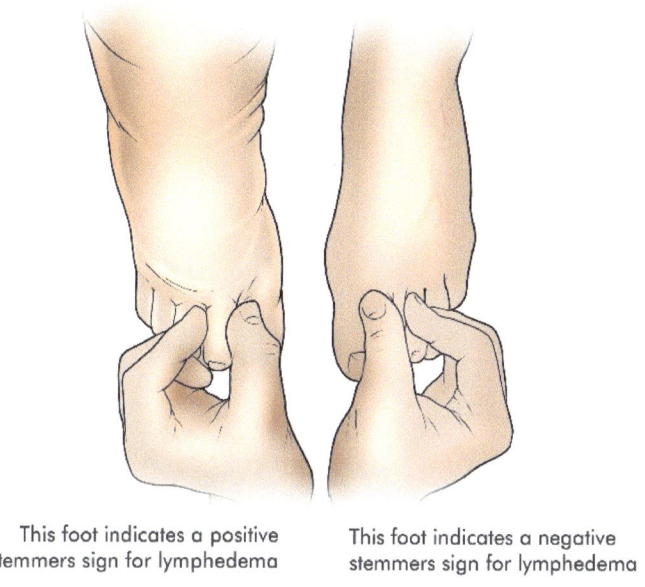

This foot indicates a positive stemmers sign for lymphedema

This foot indicates a negative stemmers sign for lymphedema

Figure 3 | A positive stemmer's sign on the right lower extremity and a negative on the left

Stages of Lymphedema

The stages of lymphedema are delineated by some key differences. Every stage of lymphedema increases the severity of symptoms, such as the skin's size, color, and texture. The more lymphedema progresses, the thicker and harder the skin becomes due to the underlying fluidic pressure. One easy way to determine if you are in stage 1 is if you notice a decrease in size and swelling in the morning after having your legs elevated all night. In addition, the early stages of lymphedema are reversible with care and management.

In contrast, the later stages of lymphedema require more intense and consistent treatment. It is critical to discuss your lymphedema with a certified lymphedema therapist to discuss your stages of lymphedema.

STAGES of LYMPHEDEMA

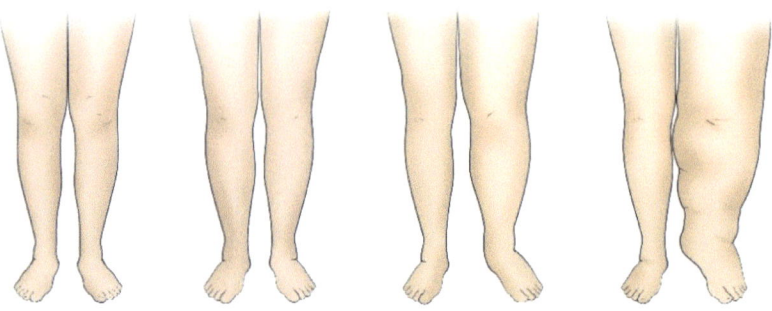

Figure 4 | The first 3 three stages of lymphedema are reversible with early intervention

Stage	Symptoms	Home Treatment	Potential Outcomes
0	No symptoms, but at risk due to known risk factors (e.g., surgery, radiation therapy)	Close monitoring and preventative measures, such as exercise and light compression socks	Reversible with preventative measures
1	Swelling and tenderness in the affected area	Node clearing, compression socks with light compression (10-20 mmHg), walking, skin care	Reversible with early intervention
2	Pronounced swelling, hardening, or thickening of the skin	Node clearing, MLD, Compression therapy with Adjustable Velcro garments (20-40mmhg), meticulous skin care, gentle exercise & walking	Reversible with intensive therapy, but may take time
3	Severe swelling, discoloration, susceptibility to infections	Node clearing, MLD, Adjustable Velcro Garments (30-50mmhg), meticulous skin care, exercise & walking, surgery in some cases	Non-reversible but can be managed with ongoing treatment

Table 1 | The stages of lymphedema and their differences

Overall, lymphedema is a chronic condition that can have a significant impact on a person's quality of life. Understanding the causes and symptoms of lymphedema is an important first step in managing the condition. While there is no cure for lymphedema, there are a few treatment options available that can help to reduce swelling and improve lymphatic function. By utilizing this book and working closely with a healthcare provider, you can develop a comprehensive treatment plan that meets your individual needs and enhances the quality of your life.

The 5 Essentials of Treating Lymphedema at Home

	Description	Specifics
Compression	Use of compression garments or bandages to reduce swelling in the affected area during the day and off at night. Garments are easily donned and doffed.	• Compression socks • Adjustable Velcro Garments • Layered Tubi-grip
Elevation	Raising the affected limb above the heart to improve lymph flow. For the upper extremity, maintain the affected limb elevated while resting utilizing a pillow.	During a flare-up, the affected limbs need to be elevated 4-6 hours per day above the heart at 60 degrees Once stable, avoid the dependent position or down position of the affected limb while resting. Elevate 35-40 degrees 2-3 hours per day
Nutrition	Having a balanced diet low in salt, processed foods, and saturated fat.	Examples of processed foods include hot dogs, chips, condiments, soda, cookies, crackers, breads, etc.
Skin Care	Regularly cleaning and moisturizing the skin to prevent infection. Using mild soaps. Be aware of the 3 signs of infection: • Heat • Red • Pain Report signs to your doctor as soon as possible.	Soaps: • Cetaphil gentle skin cleanser • Aveeno body wash skin relief Lotions: • CeraVae 5.68ph • Aveeno Daily 5.82ph • Vaseline Intensive Rescue Skin Protectant 4.3ph • Eucerin Original Dry Skin Therapy 5.97ph • Cetaphil Daily Advance Ultra Hydrating Lotion 5.65ph • Aquaphor Lotion 5.19ph
Exercises	Perform active exercises and walking, which creates a fluid pumping effect that improves lymph flow and increases circulation to affected limbs.	Self-Massage: • Node clearing of the neck, armpit, and groin. • Diaphragm breathing • Self-MLD of the affected limb. Exercises: • Walking • Active ROM of the affected limb - ankle pumps, hip flexion, shoulder shrugs.

Table 2 | The 5 essentials of treating lymphedema at home

Chapter 2: Lymphedema Self-Care Overview

Although living with lymphedema can be challenging, there are many treatments accessible to you for controlling your symptoms and improving your quality of life. Best of all, you can take control of your lymphedema at home. Let's take the five components of lymphedema care and discuss them in a little more detail.

The Importance of Healthy Weight?

As already mentioned, obesity is a contributing factor to lymphedema. And with so many Americans suffering from obesity, it is important to discuss maintaining a healthy weight to reduce the risk of developing lymphedema. People with lymphedema need to stay at a healthy weight because being overweight puts a taxing effort on the lymphatic system and makes symptoms worse. Maintaining a healthy weight and enhancing lymphatic function can be achieved by eating a balanced diet. The chapter on nutrition will go into more detail on what foods to avoid. However, there is no one specific diet for lymphedema. In general, the most beneficial diet will be a diet that has whole and unprocessed foods as the foundation. This subject can be overwhelming, and I suggest you focus on implementing one small change on a daily or weekly basis. In Chapter 5, you will find an example of a seven-day meal plan that consists of unprocessed, low-sodium, and whole foods.

Keeping the Skin Safe

Because lymphedema patients are more likely to get skin infections, skin care is crucial. Among some recommendations for skin protection are:

1. Keep your skin dry and spotless.
2. Refrain from applying harsh chemicals or soaps to your skin.
3. Apply a low-pH moisturizer.
4. Prevent skin injuries like sunburns. Check your surroundings for dangers such as sharp corners etc.
5. Use gloves, socks and/or pants when performing tasks (like gardening or cleaning) that could harm your skin.
6. Use insect repellent to prevent insect bites, which might result in skin illnesses.

Avoid Wearing Restricted Clothes

For instance, tight bras, waistbands, or jewelry may restrict lymphatic flow and aggravate symptoms. Wearing loose-fitting clothing and accessories can improve lymphatic function and minimize swelling. I advise acquiring clothing one size bigger than your typical size and made of elastic and breathable material.

The Use of Good Hygiene

People with lymphedema should practice good cleanliness because it can assist in warding off opportunistic bacterial, viral, or fungal infections. The following are some pointers for maintaining proper hygiene:

1. Regularly wash your hands to stop the transmission of germs.
2. Maintain neat and well-trimmed nails.
3. Refrain from sharing personal stuff like washcloths and towels.
4. If you find yourself in a circumstance where you cannot wash your hands, use hand sanitizer.

Exercise Frequently

Exercise is important in managing lymphedema because it helps the lymphatic system work better and reduces swelling. It's crucial to start out cautiously and build up to your desired intensity and length of exercise. I recommend you begin with 15 minutes of gentle, low-impact exercise daily and progress from there. The following are risk-free physical activities for those with lymphedema:

1. Walking
2. Swimming
3. Yoga
4. Weight training (with light weights)
5. Node clearing
   (Chapter 7 will explore in more detail exercises for the home)

Exercise is an integral part of managing lymphedema. By following these simple strategies, you can help to keep your symptoms under control and improve your quality of life. Please work closely with your healthcare provider to develop a comprehensive treatment plan that meets your individual needs.

Chapter 3: Manual Lymphatic Drainage Therapy

People with lymphedema can benefit from manual lymphatic drainage (MLD) therapy. This is a type of massage that helps to increase lymphatic flow and lessen swelling. MLD differs from traditional massage because it only applies gentle stretching pressure on the skin. The direction of the skin stretching is dictated by the body's natural lymph flow called watersheds.

How Does Manual Lymphatic Drainage Therapy Work?

Manual lymphatic drainage will increase lymphatic flow and decrease swelling in lymphedema patients. This process is referred to as decongestion. Various techniques are available such as Vodder, Foldi, and Casley Smith. These methods generally include applying a certain pattern of soft, rhythmic strokes to the skin to help lymph fluid travel through the body's watersheds.

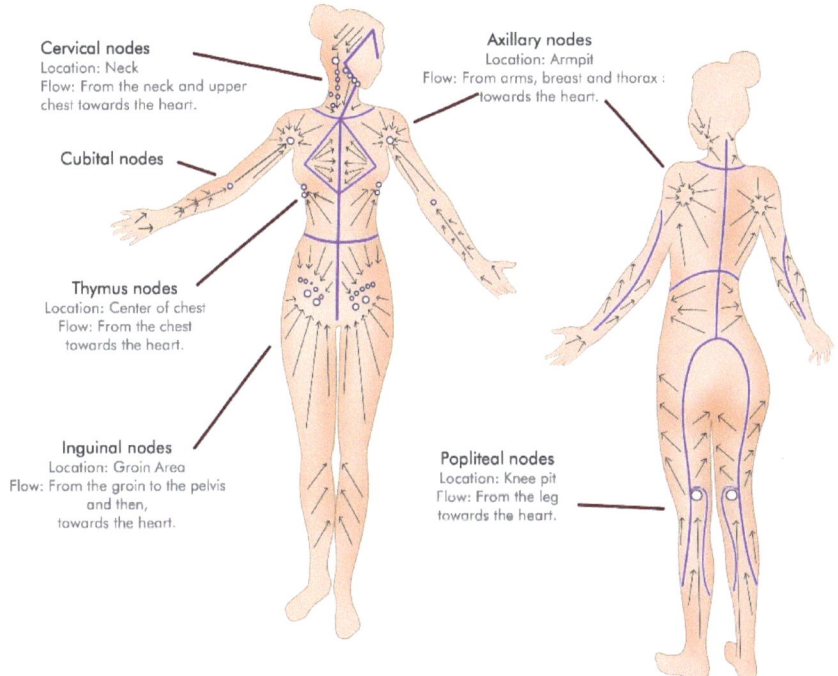

Figure 5 | The lymphatic fluid pathways called watersheds

How Effective is MLD Therapy?

By stimulating the space and skin directly above the lymphatic arteries and nodes, MLD therapy helps to improve lymphatic flow and lessen swelling. The fluid pressure in the gaps between cells can be lowered via manual lymphatic drainage (MLD). (Interstitial fluid pressure). More fluid may be able to enter lymphatic veins and be removed from the body because of the pressure drop. The lymphatic pump, a system of lymphatic tubes and valves, can also be activated by MLD. This pump makes it easier for lymphatic fluid to circulate throughout the body, which can aid in reducing edema and enhancing lymphatic circulation.

The following are just a few advantages of MLD therapy for those with lymphedema:

1. Almost immediate decrease size and swelling of affected limb.
2. Decreased pain and discomfort: MLD therapy can aid in lessening lymphedema-related pain and discomfort.
3. Increased range of motion of the affected limb
4. Decrease risk of infection
5. Stress reduction and relaxation are two benefits of MLD therapy.
6. Improve quality of life by allowing to fit into regular clothes and improve mobility.

MLD Therapy is Beneficial for Whom?

MLD treatment helps people in the middle to late stages of lymphedema, but they need to work with a certified lymphedema therapist (CLT) who understands their specific needs. MLD therapy might not be suitable for everyone, especially if you have particular health problems like active infection or blood clots.

To address lymphedema, manual lymphatic drainage therapy can be helpful. It is a secure and reliable method that can enhance lymphatic flow, lessen edema, and enhance the general quality of life. Make sure to engage with a qualified and experienced therapist who can assist you in creating a customized treatment plan if you are thinking about MLD therapy. Additionally, there are videos online that can assist you in performing a 5–8-minute upper extremity or lower extremity MLD routine at home. These routines should be performed two to three times per day. 'Self-massage for lymphedema' might be used to start a search.

Node Clearing Exercises

Prior to beginning manual lymphatic drainage, it is important to prepare the lymph nodes to receive and process fluid. This is accomplished by gently stretching the skin above the body's primary areas containing lymph nodes. Perform node clearing in a gentle and rhythmic direction, illustrated by the arrows in the diagrams below. Begin with the neck, then the armpit, and end with the groin. One easy way to remember this pattern is the acronym NAG. Node clearing can be performed on each side of the body 15 repetitions 3-5 times per day.

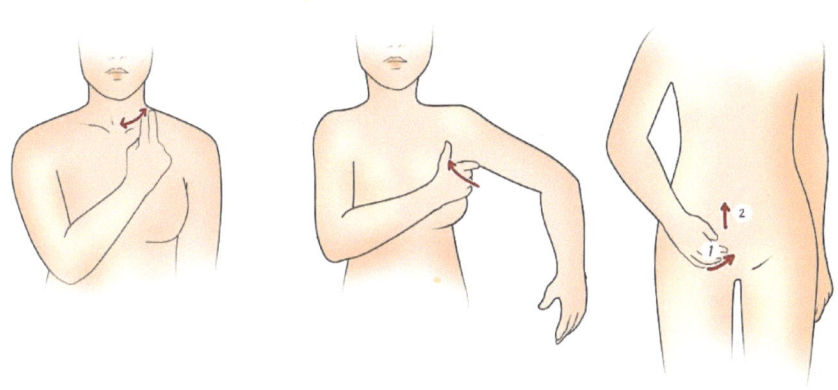

Figure 6 | Node clearing of the neck, armpit, and groin (NAG)

Diaphragmatic Breathing

Another critical aspect of preparing the body to move fluid is to perform diaphragmatic breathing exercises. There is an abundance of lymph vessels and nodes located in the trunk. Therefore, diaphragmatic breathing is an effective way to stimulate this area to move fluid. During inspiration, the diaphragm pushes down to inflate the lungs, causing the belly to stick out. During expiration, the diaphragm rises when the lungs deflate, which causes the abdomen to get sucked in. This is why diaphragmatic breathing is also called belly breathing.

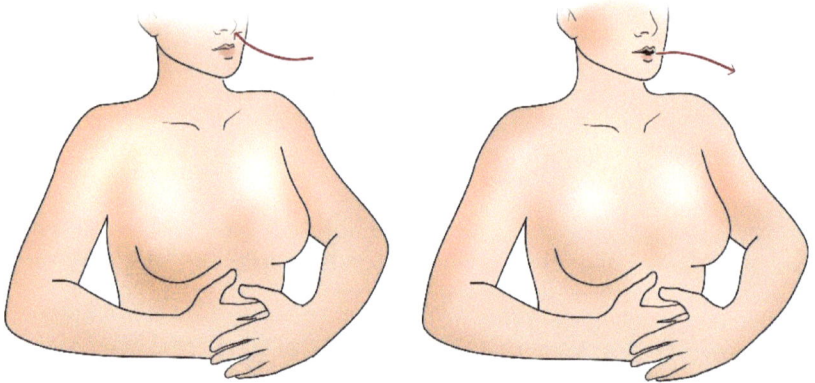

Figure 7 | Diaphragmatic/belly breathing improves the lymphatic flow of the trunk.

Chapter 4: Compression Garments

Lymphedema management requires the use of compression clothing. Compression clothing will be discussed in detail in this chapter, along with how it functions and how lymphedema sufferers can benefit from it.

What Exactly are Compression Garments?

Specialized clothing called compression garments is made to put pressure on the affected limb. They are offered in various forms, including sleeves, stockings, and gloves, and come in a range of compression levels.

How Does Compression Function?

The pressure from the garment moves lymph fluid through the lymphatic system and back into the circulatory system. Lymph fluid is propelled through lymphatic channels and back into the circulatory system due to the pressure the garment creates.

Compression garments have several advantages for lymphedema sufferers, some of which are as follows:

- Reduced edema: Wearing compression garments/socks aid in reducing edema in the affected limb.
- Improved lymphatic flow: Wearing compression garments/socks can help to increase lymphatic flow and lower the risk of lymphedema problems.
- Reduced risk of infection: Skin infections, which are frequent in lymphedema patients, can be helped by compression clothing.
- Increased mobility: Compression clothing can enhance the affected limb's movement.
- Compression garments improve balance, reduce fall risk, and enhance quality of life.
- Provide a barrier that protects the skin from damage that can be caused by interacting with the sharp surfaces of the environment.

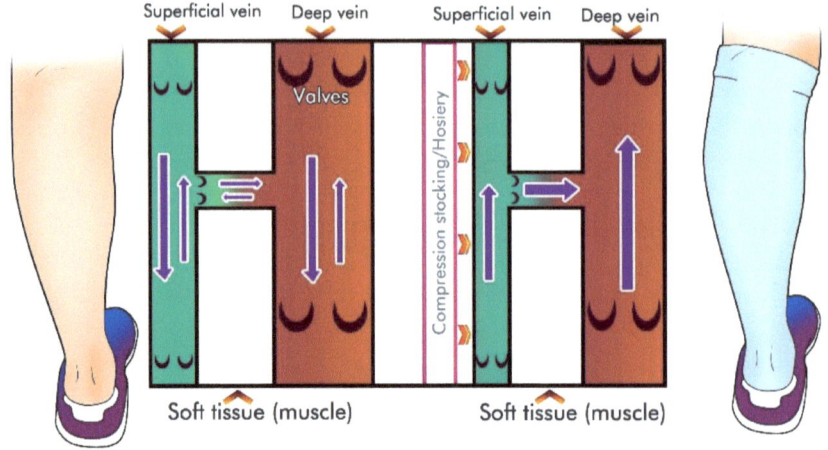

Figure 8 | When fluids are compressed, the flow rate increases

Selecting the Best Compression Garments

Choosing the appropriate compression garments is crucial to get optimal results. The garments should be well-fitting and offer the right amount of compression. Garments can be ordered off the shelf or custom, but in either case, they should be fitted by a professional. There are many reliable and high-quality manufacturers available. Sigvaris is one example of a reputable manufacturer that provides effective and high-quality garments.

Their latest catalog can be downloaded for free at:

https://www.sigvaris.com/en-us/our-services/download-center/download-catalog-lookbooks

There are two types of compression clothing to think about for self-care. Compression stockings and adjustable Velcro garments are the best options when considering self-care in the home. Both garment types have advantages and disadvantages.

Recommended Compression Garments and Description	Pros	Cons
Adjustable Velcro Garments: Provide adjustable compression more appropriate during flare-ups and later stages of lymphedema when more containment is needed. Sigvaris Compreflex products. I recommend an additional transitional liner for the lower extremity.	Sturdy, adjustable fit, easy to use	Expensive, impermeable
Stockings with Compression: Provide non-adjustable static compression that is more appropriate in earlier stages of lymphedema. Sigvaris offers different colors and fabrics that best suit your needs. Sigvaris also offers multiple devices that can aid in donning and doffing.	Affordable, lightweight, breathable	Not adjustable, not sturdy, difficult to put on/take off

Table 3 | Compression options for self-care at home

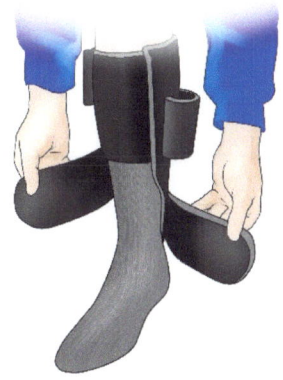
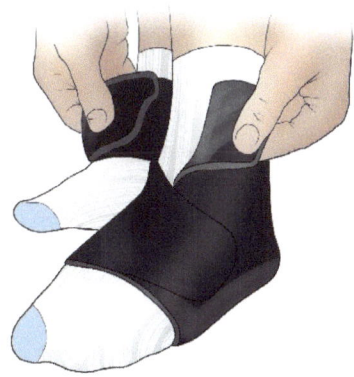

Figure 9 | Adjustable Velcro garments - the best option for flare-ups and daily care at home

Please get advice from a licensed therapist with lymphedema certification to establish the ideal level of compression required for your circumstance. Typically, you start with a lesser compression (10-20mmhg) in the early stages of lymphedema. During flare-ups or later stages of lymphedema, you can gradually increase the compression level to 20 to 40 mmHg to accommodate changes as the affected area shrinks in size and swelling.

Maintaining Compression Garments

The effectiveness of compression garments depends on proper maintenance. Each manufacturer provides their own specific guidelines. In general, compression garments should be laundered frequently. They should not be put in the dryer; instead, they should be hung to dry.

Overall, an essential component of treating lymphedema is wearing compression clothing. They can aid in reducing edema, enhancing lymphatic circulation, and improving the general quality of life. Work with a healthcare provider or qualified fitter if you're considering wearing compression clothing so they can advise you on the best option and ensure it fits you properly.

Chapter 5: Nutrition and Lymphedema

Since lymphedema is a chronic disorder, continual care is necessary to prevent symptoms. Although there is no known cure for lymphedema, some lifestyle choices, like diet and stress reduction, can significantly impact how symptoms are managed.

The Role of Nutrition in Lymphedema Management

What we eat can significantly impact how our bodies work, including how they manage fluid balance. A nutritious diet high in protein and fiber and low in sodium can aid persons with lymphedema by reducing swelling and inflammation. Following are some dietary suggestions for controlling lymphedema:

1. **Limit your salt intake** to decrease water retention, which worsens lymphedema symptoms. Avoid processed foods high in sodium and experiment with herbs and spices to flavor your food instead of salt to lower your salt intake. 'Green Salt' is an excellent natural alternative to traditional salt. It is a plant-based substitute made from dehydrated Salicornia.
2. **Increase your protein intake**: Protein helps the body create and repair tissues. Lean meats, fish, eggs, and beans are examples of foods high in protein that can assist in minimizing swelling and promote efficient lymphatic function.
3. **Increase your fiber intake**: Fiber is essential for preventing constipation, which can put stress on the lymphatic system and promote regular bowel movements. Consuming meals high in fiber, such as whole grains, fruits, and vegetables, can assist in keeping things moving.

There isn't a set recommendation for salt intake when dealing with lymphedema. Generally, you will need to reduce your salt intake to lessen the body's tendency to swell brought on by salt. In addition, decrease the consumption of highly processed foods; often, these are long-lasting items that come in a box, bag, or container. The lymphatic system must work harder to process and eliminate the additives in these foods.

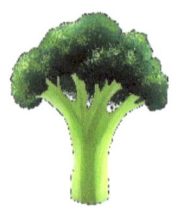

I have compiled a list of foods that are the most highly processed, along with their approximate sodium content:

Most highly processed foods	Sodium Content per Serving
Fast food	1,000-2,500 mg
Packaged snacks	100-300 mg
Sweetened beverages	<200 mg
Frozen meals	500-1,500 mg
Instant noodles	Up to 2,000 mg
Breakfast cereals	100-300 mg
Processed meats	Up to 400 mg
Microwave popcorn	Up to 300 mg
Margarine	Up to 200 mg
Condiments (e.g., ketchup, mayonnaise)	Up to 150 mg
Salad dressing	Up to 350 mg
Potato chips	120-180 mg
Gravy	140-290 mg

Table 4 | The most common processed foods

Lifestyle Variables Affecting Lymphedema Symptoms

Various lifestyle variables might affect lymphedema symptoms in addition to diet. Here are some factors to consider:

1. Stress: The hormone cortisol, which can raise inflammation and fluid retention, is one that stress can make the body generate. Deep breathing exercises, yoga, meditation, and other stress-reduction techniques can assist in lessening the symptoms of increased cortisol.
2. Smoking: It can cause the body to become more inflammatory, worsening lymphedema symptoms. Inflammation can be decreased by giving up smoking.
3. Alcohol: Drinking alcohol can cause the body to become dehydrated, which can make lymphedema symptoms worse. Consuming alcohol in moderation can help manage symptoms.

In order to effectively manage lymphedema, a holistic strategy that considers medical care, lifestyle variables, and dietary considerations are necessary. You may actively manage your lymphedema symptoms and enhance your general health by being mindful of what you eat and how you conduct your life.

The Importance of Hydration and Lymphedema

There is no specific guideline for water intake for those suffering from lymphedema. However, in general, drinking half an ounce to one ounce of water for every pound of body weight is recommended. For example, if you weigh 200 pounds, you should consume 100 to 200 ounces of water per day. The amount of daily activity, the temperature of the environment, age, and sex also play an important part in water intake. The more active you are, the more water your body needs to sustain healthy lymphatic function.

One way to find a registered dietician in your area, either in person or via telehealth, is to visit https://www.eatright.org/find-a-nutrition-expert

Strategies for Water Intake	Recommended Daily Water Intake
General Guidelines	64 ounces (8 cups) per day
Body weight	Half an ounce to one ounce of water per pound of body weight per day
Physical activity	Active individuals may need to increase their water intake
Environment	Increase water intake in hot or dry climates
Gender	2.7 liters (91 ounces) per day for adult women and 3.7 liters (125 ounces) per day for adult men, including water from all sources

Table 5 | Strategies for water intake at home

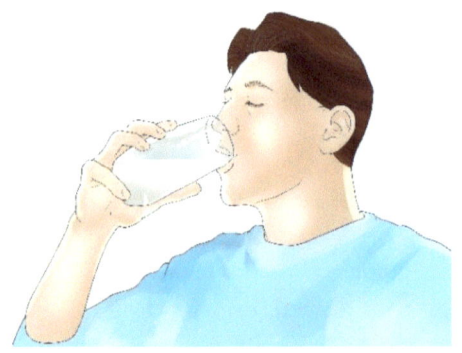

Figure 10 | There are several strategies for water intake at home

The following are two examples of a 7-day meal plans that have very low sodium and eliminates processed foods. The first meal plan has almost no sodium and can be used when your lymphedema has flared up, and you are heavily retaining fluid. The second meal plan contains low to moderate sodium and should be sustained all year round.

Please note that these are only meant to be an example, and everyone's additional needs vary. In general, to effectively manage lymphedema at home, you must always maintain a low-sodium diet.

Day	Breakfast	Snack	Lunch	Snack	Dinner	Total Sodium (mg)
1	1/2 cup steel-cut oats (0 mg)	1 small apple (0 mg)	3 oz grilled chicken breast (50 mg)	1 medium carrot (42 mg)	3 oz baked salmon with 3 oz roasted asparagus (30 mg)	122
2	1 slice whole wheat toast (90 mg)	1/2 small banana (0 mg)	3 oz lentil soup (35 mg)	1 small pear (0 mg)	3 oz grilled chicken breast with 3 oz steamed broccoli (35 mg)	160
3	1/2 cup steel-cut oats (0 mg)	1 small carrot (42 mg)	3 oz grilled turkey breast (50 mg)	1 small apple (0 mg)	3 oz baked cod with 3 oz steamed Brussels sprouts (45 mg)	137
4	3/4 cup plain non-fat Greek yogurt (35 mg)	1/2 small peach (0 mg)	3 oz low-sodium canned tuna (45 mg)	1 small carrot (42 mg)	3 oz grilled flank steak with 3 oz sautéed kale (50 mg)	172
5	1/2 cup egg whites (55 mg)	1 small apple (0 mg)	3 oz grilled chicken breast (50 mg)	1 hard-boiled egg white (10 mg)	3 oz broiled cod with 3 oz roasted asparagus (20 mg)	135
6	3/4 cup low-fat cottage cheese (225 mg)	1 small peach (0 mg)	3 oz grilled portobello mushroom (20 mg)	1/2 small pineapple (0 mg)	3 oz baked salmon with 3 oz steamed green beans (50 mg)	295 mg
7	1/2 cup steel-cut oats (0 mg)	1/4 cup raw almonds (0 mg)	3 oz lentil soup (35 mg)	3 oz non-fat Greek yogurt (35 mg)	3 oz grilled chicken breast with 3 oz roasted Brussels sprouts (75 mg)	180 mg

Table 6 | Example of an ultra-low sodium 7-day meal plan used during flare-ups

Day	Breakfast	Snack	Lunch	Snack	Dinner	Total Sodium (mg)
1	Quinoa and Berry Breakfast Bowl (4 oz, 140 mg)	Apple slices with almond butter (1 oz, 0 mg)	Grilled Chicken Salad (4 oz, 130 mg)	Raw veggies with hummus (2 oz, 35 mg)	Baked salmon w/ roasted asparagus and sweet potato (4 oz, 65 mg)	470
2	Whole wheat toast with avocado and sliced tomato (2 oz, 100 mg)	Greek yogurt w/ mixed berries and chopped walnuts (6 oz, 65 mg)	Lentil and Vegetable Soup (8 oz, 55 mg)	Fresh pear (1 oz, 0 mg)	Grilled chicken breast, steamed broccoli, and brown rice (4 oz, 50 mg)	370
3	Oatmeal, banana, and almond butter (8 oz, 0 mg)	Raw veggies with hummus (2 oz, 35 mg)	Turkey and Swiss Cheese Sandwich (4 oz, 200 mg)	Fresh apple slices (1 oz, 0 mg)	Baked cod w/ Brussels sprouts and quinoa (4 oz, 65 mg)	400
4	Greek yogurt, mixed berries, chopped walnuts (6 oz, 65 mg)	Fresh peach (1 oz, 0 mg)	Tuna Salad Lettuce Wraps (4 oz, 155 mg)	Raw veggies with hummus (2 oz, 35 mg)	Grilled flank steak w/ sautéed kale and roasted sweet potato (4 oz, 65 mg)	420
5	Veggie Omelet (4 oz, 140 mg)	Apple slices with almond butter (1 oz, 0 mg)	Grilled Chicken Salad (4 oz, 160 mg)	Hard-boiled egg (2 oz, 70 mg)	Broiled Cod w/ roasted asparagus and quinoa (4 oz, 30 mg)	500
6	Cottage Cheese w/ sliced peaches and sliced almonds (6 oz, 85 mg)	Baby Carrots with guacamole (2 oz, 50 mg)	Portobello Mushroom Sandwich (4 oz, 105 mg)	Fresh Pineapple chunks (1 oz, 0 mg)	Baked Salmon w/ steamed green beans and roasted red potatoes (4 oz, 60 mg)	385
7	Rolled Oats with mixed berries, sliced almonds, and non-fat milk (8 oz, 80 mg)	Raw almonds (1 oz, 0 mg)	Lentil Soup w/ mixed greens salad (8 oz, 150 mg)	Non-fat Greek yogurt with sliced strawberries (6 oz, 35 mg)	Grilled Chicken Breast with roasted Brussels sprouts and brown rice (4 oz, 75 mg)	440

Table 7 | Example of a low sodium 7-day meal plan that can be maintained all year around

Chapter 6: Skin Care and Lymphedema

Maintaining good skin health is essential for managing lymphedema. The primary purpose of skin care for lymphedema is to prevent harmful infections. As a result of the fluid buildup brought on by lymphedema, your skin undergoes increased pressure which compromises its integrity. Therefore, you will be more prone to opportunistic infections. We'll talk about the value of daily checks, how to correctly wash your skin and the application of low-pH moisturizers and skin care equipment.

Skin Examinations Every Day

Daily skin examinations are crucial to lymphedema management. Look for any variations in tightness, color, or temperature as well as indications of infection, including heat, redness, or pain (HRP). Contact your healthcare practitioner straight away if you detect any changes. For a complete inspection, you can also use a long-handle mirror and flashlight on hard-to-see areas or skin folds.

Suitable Skin Washing

Use lukewarm water and a gentle, fragrance-free soap to wash your skin. Hot water and abrasive soaps can irritate the skin and make lymphedema symptoms worse. Avoid rubbing or scrubbing your skin as you gently pat it dry with a soft cloth. Here are some instances of mild skin soaps.

1. Gentle Skin Cleanser by Cetaphil
2. Body Wash Aveeno Skin Relief

Application of Low-pH Moisturizer

Maintaining the skin's natural acidity and shielding it from irritation can both be accomplished by using a moisturizer with a low ph. Look for a moisturizer that is intended specifically for sensitive skin and is fragrance-free. Here are a few examples of low-pH lotions to manage lymphedema at home.

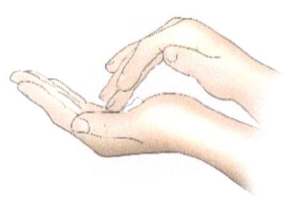

Lotion Name	pH Level
CeraVae	5.68
Aveeno Daily Skin Relief	5.82
Vaseline Intensive Rescue	4.3
Eucerin Original Dry Skin Therapy	5.97
Cetaphil Daily Advance Hydrating	5.65
Aquaphor Lotion	5.19

Table 8 | Low-pH lotions

Skin Care Tool	Function
Sponge with a long handle	Assists in reaching lower legs and feet when bathing
Reacher with a long handle	Assists in reaching objects on the floor.
Manicure tool	For maintaining healthy nails
Long-reach toenail scissors	For maintaining healthy nails
Lotion spray or roll-on	Aquaphor has a spray-on option making daily moisturizing easier
Leg lifter	To assist with the daily elevation of legs onto an ottoman or bed.
Portable shower head	Allows washing a larger surface area of the skin.
Shower stool	Allows a person to sit in the shower, thus creating a safer environment
Sock Aide	Assists in donning socks without bending.
Dressing rod	Assists with donning pants without the need for bending.

Table 9 | Assistive skin care and dressing tools for self-care at home

You may help prevent skin issues, infections, and maintain healthy, moisturized skin while managing lymphedema by including these skin care practices into your regular regimen.

Chapter 7: Exercise and Lymphedema

Exercise is one of the fundamental essentials in managing lymphedema at home. Think of exercise as taking medicine for a chronic condition, except your prescription has infinite refills. The prescription for lymphedema exercises is twice per day for just 5-10 minutes.

Advantages of Exercise

Exercise can help with edema reduction, lymphatic function improvement, and general physical and mental health improvement. While resistance training can help build muscle and improve strength, aerobic activity, such as walking, range of motion, or swimming, can enhance lymphatic flow and circulation. Yoga and stretching will also benefit your flexibility and range of motion.

Safety Measures for Exercise

While exercise can help lymphedema, some measures should be taken to prevent aggravating the illness. These safety measures could include:

- Putting on compression clothing while working out to help minimize edema.
- Begin slowly and progressively increase the duration and intensity of your activity.
    - Start with 5-10 repetitions on both sides of your body twice per day and gradually increase to 10-20 repetitions on both sides three times per day.
- Refraining from actions that could place the affected limb under undue strain. For example, avoid excessive straining or using equipment that can damage the skin.
- Stopping physical activity if you feel pain, discomfort, or swelling increases.

Additionally, speaking with a CLT before beginning an exercise regimen is crucial, particularly if you have advanced or severe lymphedema.

Tips for Exercise for Lymphedema

There are several guidelines to remember when exercising while dealing with lymphedema to ensure efficiency and safety. These pointers might include:

- Maintaining hydration to support lymphatic flow. (See Table 5)
- Including a low-impact aerobic activity in your program, such as range of motion or walking
- Engaging in resistance training with light weights and high repetitions while avoiding activities that place an undue amount of strain on the affected limb(s)
- Using a brush or massage ball to ease tension and encourage lymphatic movement.
- Including yoga and stretching to increase flexibility and ease tension.

Exercise Type for Lymphedema	Examples	Repetitions	Frequency	Precautions
Breathing	Diaphragmatic exercises, deep breathing, Counting breathing	5 times	2-3x per day	May cause lightheadedness
Upper Extremity	Shoulder shrugs, neck rolls, shoulder abduction, elbow curls, wrist curls, fist pumps.	15-20 reps on both sides	2-3 x per day	Avoid the affected side if it causes pain.
Lower Extremity	Ankle pumps, knee extension, knee flexion, hip extension, straight leg raise, hip abduction.	15-20 repetitions	2-3 x per day	Perform slowly in a seated position or lying on a bed
Trunk	Flexion, extension, abdominal contractions, side bending	15-20 repetitions	2-3 x per day	Perform in a seated or standing position.

Table 10 | Fundamental home exercises for lymphedema self-care at home

Home Exercise Program for Lymphedema

Perform all exercises 10-15 times on each side of the body twice per day.

Figure 11 | Home Exercise Program (HEP) for daily maintenance of lymphedema

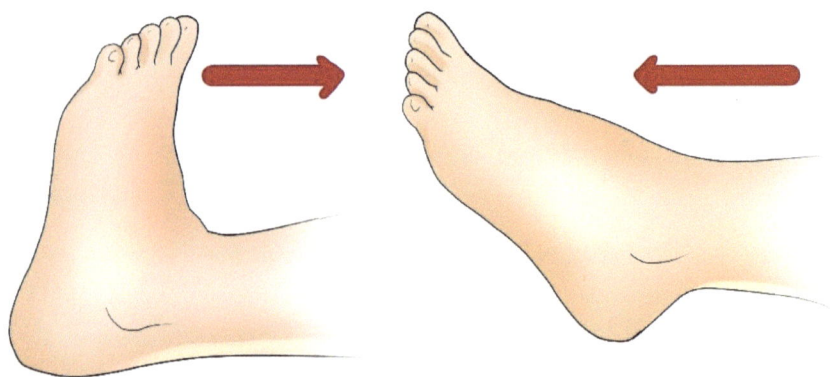

1. **Ankle Pump** - *pump the ankle up and down slowly*

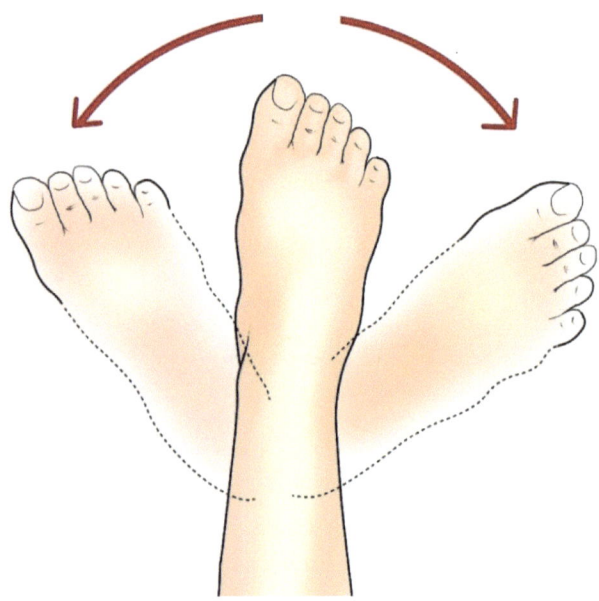

2. **Ankle Circles** - *make a circle slowly*

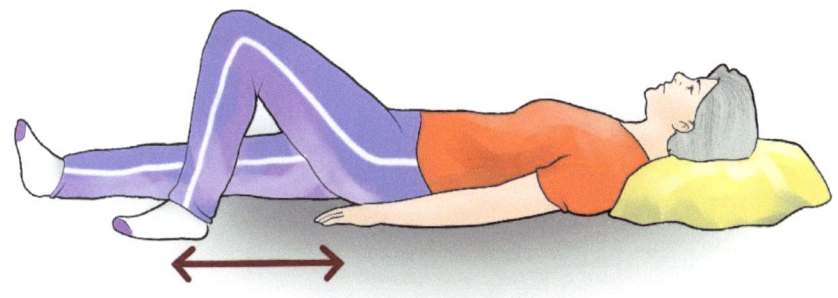

*3. **Heel Slides** - slide the heels up and down slowly*

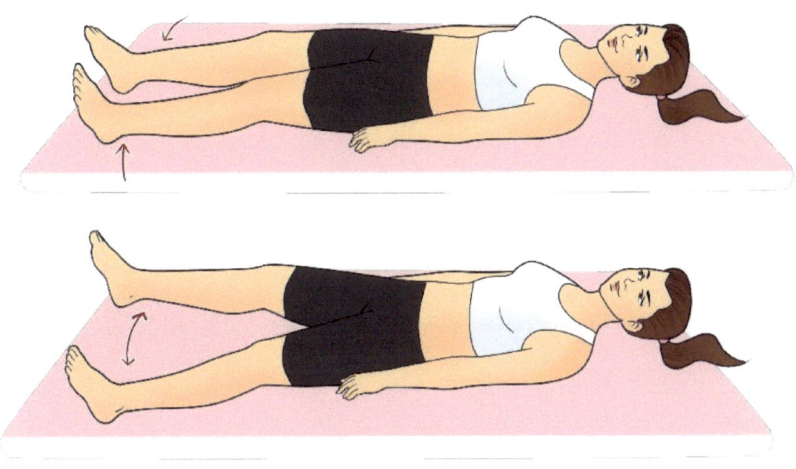

*4. **Leg Slides** - slide your legs like scissors slowly*

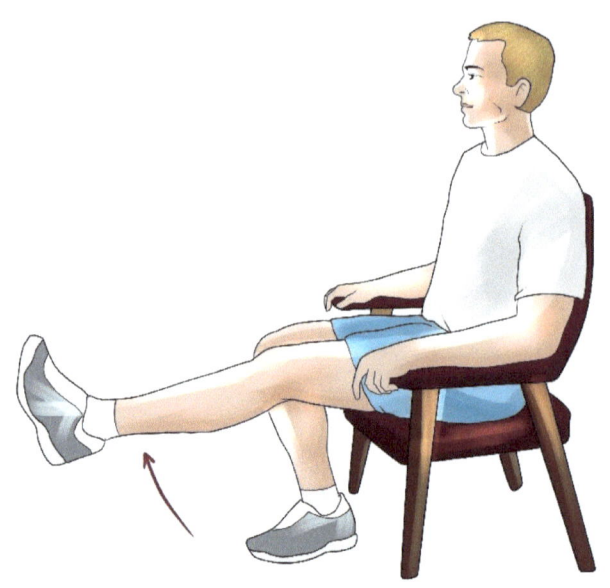

5. **Knee Extension** - *kick leg up and down slowly*

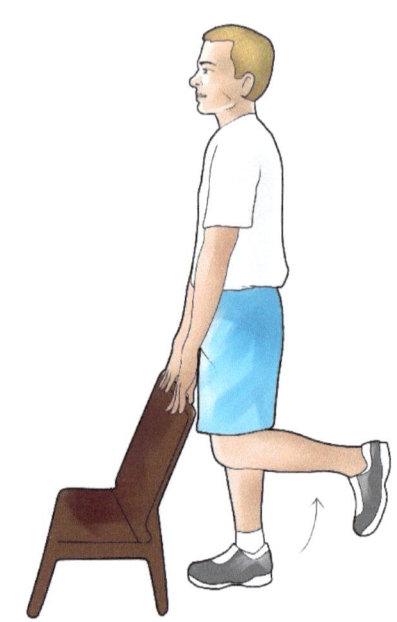

6. **Knee Flexion** - *bend your knee up and down*

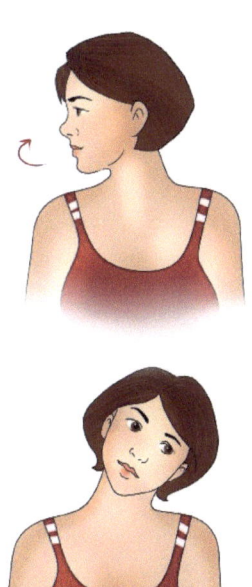

*7. **Neck Turning** - turn the head slowly*

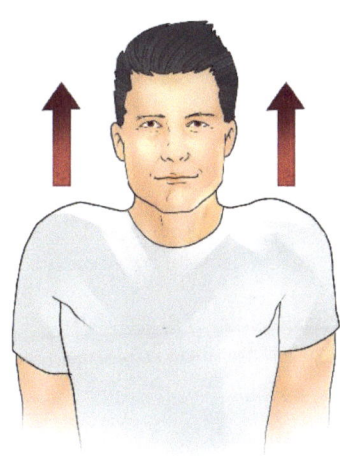

*8. **Shoulder Shrugs** - lift shoulders up and down slowly*

Why do all my therapists recommend walking as the best exercise for lymphedema?

The answer is simple. Walking is an excellent exercise because it causes a pumping effect in the calf muscle, as illustrated below. This calf muscle pump assists in improving circulation to the lower extremities, which reduces swelling. Furthermore, walking with compression garments on compounds the pumping action of the calf and improves circulation even more.

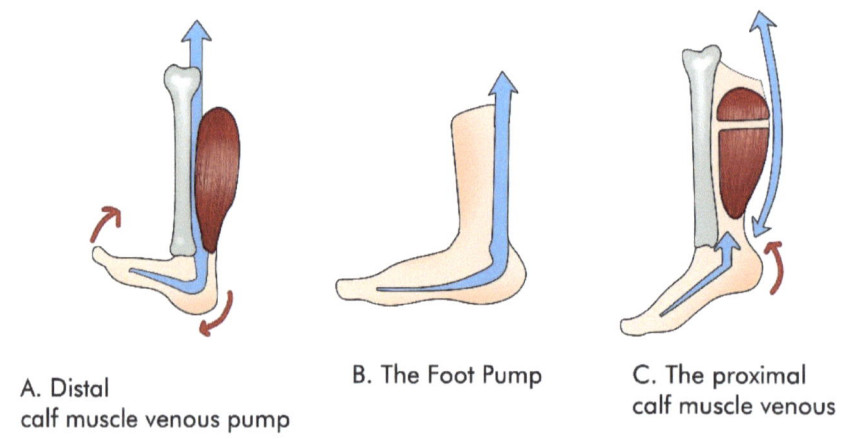

A. Distal calf muscle venous pump

B. The Foot Pump

C. The proximal calf muscle venous

Figure 12 | Walking creates a calf muscle pump for lower extremity lymphatic flow

Exercise can help manage lymphedema, but it's vital to take safety measures and talk to your doctor or therapist before beginning an exercise regimen. You can enhance lymphatic function and general physical and mental health while dealing with lymphedema by including low-impact aerobic activity, weight training, stretching, and mindfulness into your regimen.

When you work with a specialist in person, they can provide guidance and accountability during all stages of care. At home, this book can provide the guidance you need. Accountability is difficult when working alone. Remember, I offer telehealth visits if you reach out to me on social media to schedule an accountability coaching session. For now, I am challenging you to use the checklist I have provided for 30 days and start holding yourself accountable. We can face the challenges together, but I still need your participation. Do your best – that is all I ask.

Chapter 8: Elevation

What Happens During Elevation?

The lymphatic system is not a one-man show. In fact, it is responsible for up to 15% of your body's circulation. When you have lymphedema, it is essential to elevate the affected limb often. Fluids are removed from the area when a limb is lifted, which enhances circulation and lowers swelling. To pump fluids and blood against gravity, the body must exert more effort, which improves circulation generally and puts less strain on the heart. Depending on the problem's severity, different levels of elevation may be advised for lymphedema therapy.

Elevating the affected leg is crucial for lowering swelling and treating symptoms when lymphedema flares up. During a flare-up, I advise you to elevate the affected limb to an elevation of at least 60 degrees above the heart. This encourages enhanced lymphatic fluid outflow and circulation in the afflicted area. I recommend six hours per day spread throughout the day during flare-ups. When your limbs resume their normal size, you can decrease the elevation time. The proper level of elevation during a flare-up should be determined in consultation with a healthcare expert because it may vary depending on the demands and conditions of the individual.

Elevation therapy for lymphedema management must be consistently practiced for long-term results. For the best outcome, continue elevating the legs for 3 hours per day at an angle of 30-45 degrees. The more inactive or stationary you are, the more lymphedema tends to rise. Maintaining a constant elevation may also aid in promoting steady lymphatic fluid drainage and preventing the buildup of extra fluid. Whether you're flared up or stable, your affected limbs should be propped up on a pillow or ottoman when resting.

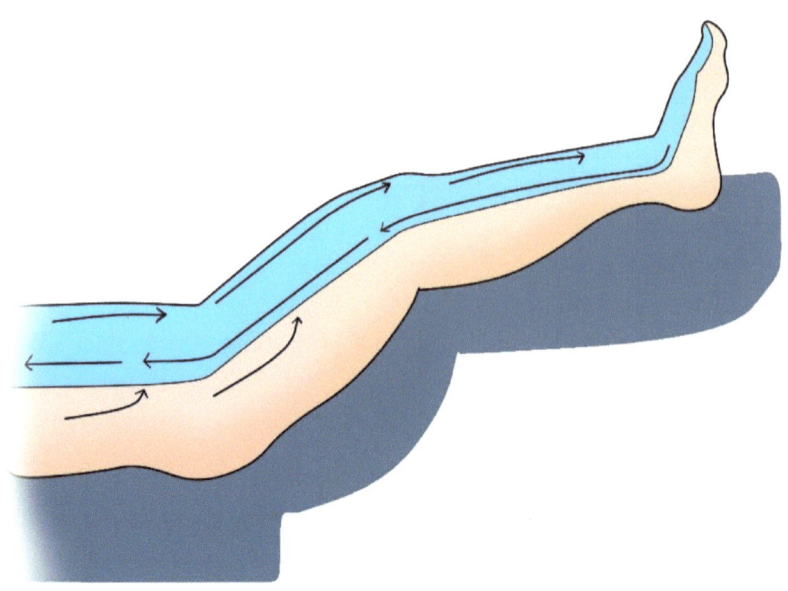

Figure 13 | Elevation is an essential part of lymphedema self-care at home

Chapter 9: Traveling with Lymphedema

Tips for Comfortable and Safe Travel

Advice for plane travel and lengthy automobile rides while traveling with lymphedema:

It's crucial to take precautions to maintain comfort and safety when traveling with lymphedema. It's important to wear compression clothing when flying, and you might want to think about asking for an aisle seat so you can move around easily and stretch. While traveling, it is important to take regular breaks to improve circulation to the affected limb. During these breaks, you should walk, perform ankle pumps, and do gentle stretching.

Travel Safety Precautions and Precautions to Take

While traveling with lymphedema, taking care of your skin is crucial to avoid damage or infection. This includes avoiding constrictive clothes or jewelry, drinking enough water, and taking precautions to prevent insect bites or sunburns, which can raise the risk of infection.

How to be Ready for Unexpected Situations While Traveling

It's crucial to prepare for emergencies when traveling with lymphedema. The following table illustrates a few examples of supplies to bring with you when traveling. You should also consider carrying any necessary equipment, such as compression garments or pumps. Additionally, it's a good idea to investigate the nearby medical facilities in case of an emergency and carry your healthcare providers' information.

Supplies to Bring When Traveling with Lymphedema	Purpose
Adjustable Velcro Garments	Provide compression and support for affected areas
Compression pump	Maintain lymphatic flow and reduce swelling
Moisturizer	Hydrate and prevent irritation of dry, itchy skin
Wipes with an antibacterial agent	Clean cuts or scrapes to prevent infection
Insect repellent	Shield the skin from insect bites and prevent infection
Sunscreen	Protect the skin from sunburn and reduce the risk of infection
Comfortable clothing and footwear	Avoid constrictive clothing and footwear and promote comfort and support
Medical alert bracelet	Provide information about your condition in case of emergency

Table 11 | Essentials for traveling with lymphedema

Remember, it's crucial to discuss any needs or concerns you may have with your CLT before traveling while experiencing lymphedema.

Chapter 10: Preventing and Managing Lymphedema Re-congestion or Flare-Ups

Lymphedema is persistent and can result in swelling in many body locations, including the arms, legs, trunk, or face. When the lymphatic system, which oversees eliminating waste and fluid from the body, is damaged or not operating properly, edema develops. Even though late-stage lymphedema can't be cured, it can be treated, and flare-ups can be reversed.

Lymphedema Triggers

Numerous things, such as an infection, an injury, surgery, or radiation therapy, can cause lymphedema. Flare-ups can also be brought on by certain activities like flying or physically demanding exercise. It's critical to be aware of these triggers and take precautions to stop lymphedema from getting worse. Sudden changes in diet can also trigger flare-ups. I have witnessed patients reverse their early-stage lymphedema only to regress due to minor changes in diet. Be consistent, diligent, and take control!

How to Prevent Re-congestion or Flare-ups

Self-care and medical treatment must be used together to keep lymphedema from getting worse or getting congested again. Self-care practices that can help avoid lymphedema include:

- Refrain from wearing jewelry or tight clothing that could restrict lymphatic movement.
- Upkeep of a healthy weight
- Whenever possible, keep the affected limb elevated. Avoid the dependent position or limb in the down position.
- Refraining from actions that could put the affected limb under undue strain, such as heavy lifting or repetitive motions.

Wearing compression garments, self-node clearing, or employing pneumatic compression devices are all possible options during a flare-up. Choosing the appropriate management strategy for flare-ups requires close collaboration with a healthcare professional. However, the five essentials of lymphedema care at home will never change. They are the cornerstone of effective lymphedema management.

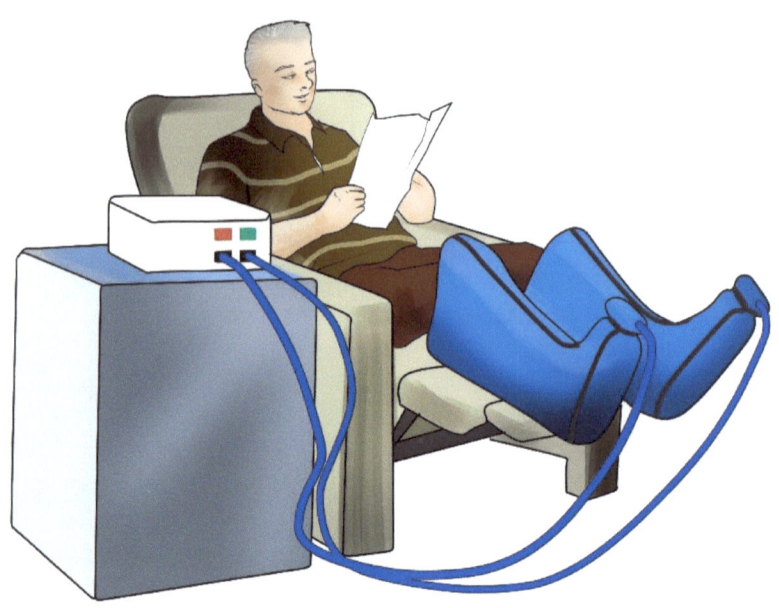

Figure 14 | Pneumatic compression pumps - an effective way to safely manage lymphedema

What to Do Right Away When Lymphedema Flares-up

When lymphedema flares-up, it's critical to act quickly to control the swelling and avoid progressive complications such as pain and skin breaks that cause weeping or infections.

Among the actions to take are:

- Raising the affected limb over the heart (See chapter 8)
- Refraining from activities that could worsen the edema, such as prolonged standing or sitting.
- Using painkillers as necessary
- Checking with a medical professional to see if antibiotics are required to prevent infection.

Adjustable Velcro Garments will be the most practical choice when treating lymphedema at home during a flare-up or re-congestion. That is because they provide a form of compression that can be easily adjusted gradually as your leg begins to decongest or decrease in size.

Making a Lymphedema First Aid Emergency Kit

Additionally, it's crucial to put together a lymphedema first aid emergency kit in case of a flare-up. Essential supplies for managing swelling and preventing infection should be included in this kit. The following things should be in a lymphedema emergency kit:

Lymphedema Emergency Supply Kit	Description
Adjustable Velcro Garments	These are important for managing flare-ups and providing support to the affected area.
Antibiotic cream	This can be used to treat or prevent infection.
Medi-Honey/Antibiotic Ointment	This natural anti-microbial and anti-inflammatory agent can also help with wound healing.
4 by 4 gauze/Rolled gauze	This is used to clean and cover wounds.
Adhesive tape	This is used to secure bandages and gauze in place.
ABD pads/Absorbent Sanitary pads	These can be used to control weeping and provide cushioning for the affected area.
Ice pack	This can be used to reduce swelling and provide pain relief.
Thermometer	A fever could be an early sign of an infection
Aspirin or another anti-fever medication	This can help to reduce fever and relieve pain.
Gloves	These are important for maintaining hygiene and preventing infection during wound care.

Table 12 | Lymphedema emergency supply kit

Along with these, it's crucial to speak with a doctor about keeping a prescription on hand in case of flare-ups or when the first indications of infection appear. Antibiotics or other drugs to treat lymphedema symptoms may be part of this prescription.

Overall, self-care practices and medical management must be used in conjunction to control lymphedema. Individuals with lymphedema can enhance their quality of life and lower their risk of problems by learning the causes of the condition and adopting precautions to stop flare-ups or re-congestion. Additionally, it is crucial to have a first aid kit on hand in case of an emergency and to speak with a medical professional for advice on treating the symptoms of lymphedema.

Chapter 11: Dealing with Minor Skin Breaks and Tears at Home

Preventing Skin Breaks and Early Detection

Maintaining good skin care while controlling lymphedema at home is crucial for avoiding skin tears or breaks. You can avoid most breaks by keeping your compression on when you're most active and being alert to your surroundings. This means keeping the area you occupy the most clean and free of sharp objects or corners. However, even if you take all the necessary precautions, accidents can happen, or mistakes can be made. Remember to inspect your skin daily; if you see any weeping, unusual swelling, or pain, these could all be signs of a skin break. Please refer to Table 12 in Chapter 10 for a complete list of what to always have on hand when living with lymphedema.

How to Clean and Bandage Minor Skin Breaks

When you have lymphedema, a small cut, tear, or break in the skin requires immediate attention to prevent infection and further damage. It's important to understand that a small tear or break can quickly turn into a situation requiring professional medical attention. Therefore, be diligent and consistent until the break, tear, or cut is fully healed. Use antibacterial soap to clean the affected area every 24 hours. If you observe the affected area to be weeping or draining fluid, then clean and cover the area every 12 hours. Beyond the first two days, avoid first-aid cleaners like hydrogen peroxide, which can delay the healing process. After cleaning the area, apply antibiotic ointment or Medi-honey, then cover the area with square gauze and an absorbing pad if there is drainage. Keep the area bandaged up until it has healed completely, and keep applying compression as usual day and night.

Compression During the Healing Process

Adjustable Velcro garments are ideal for controlling lymphedema because they allow you to customize the pressure applied to the affected area. Keep the compression on even while you sleep; it will speed up the healing process. Compression garments can be worn again only during the day once the skin has recovered.

Preventing Another Skin Break

After the skin has healed, it is important to monitor its condition to ensure it doesn't break out again. To keep your skin clean and nourished, use a mild soap and a moisturizer with a low pH (see Table 6). Taking care of your skin and preventing further consequences from lymphedema is critical, as even slight breaches in skin integrity can pose a serious threat to lymphedema patients. Following these guidelines can help you properly handle minor skin breaks and help you take control of your lymphedema at home.

Chapter 12: Common Lymphedema Complications

Lymphedema sufferers are at increased risk for developing infections like lymphangitis and cellulitis. We'll go through strategies for dealing with these problems, as well as what to do if an infection sets in.

Cellulitis

Cellulitis is one of the most common infections associated with lymphedema. This is a bacterial infection of the skin and subcutaneous tissue. Heat, redness, and pain are a few of the cellulitis symptoms and indicators (HRP). You can use the abbreviation HRP, which stands for heat, redness, and pain, to recall these symptoms. Searching for **H**igh-**R**isk **P**atterns of **H**eat, **R**edness, and **P**ain is another technique to remember.

It's critical to respond right away if you suspect cellulitis. The initial phases entail:

- **Take antibiotics**: The doctor will prescribe antibiotics if cellulitis is determined to exist. Even if your symptoms improve, make sure to finish the entire course of antibiotics as directed by the doctor. The most prescribed antibiotics for lymphedema-related skin infections include the following:
  1. **Cephalosporins**: such as cephalexin, are used for skin infections that are more severe or resistant to other antibiotics.
  2. **Trimethoprim-sulfamethoxazole**: is a combination antibiotic used to treat a variety of bacterial infections, including skin infections.
- **Elevate and rest the affected limb**: This will assist in lessening swelling and discomfort in the affected limb.
- **Use over-the-counter pain relievers** to help with pain management and fever reduction. Examples of over-the-counter pain relievers are acetaminophen and ibuprofen.
- **Hydrate well**: Hydrating well can help prevent dehydration, which can exacerbate symptoms.

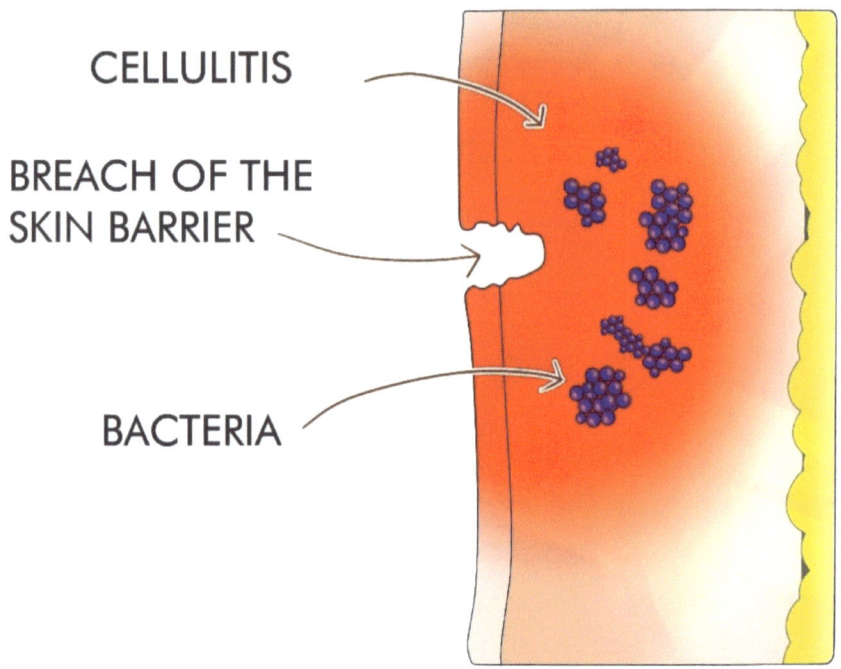

Figure 15 | Cellulitis is caused by even a minor breach in skin integrity

Lymphangitis

Another problem connected to lymphedema is lymphangitis. This lymphatic artery infection can cause fever, chills, and general malaise. Remember to look for the *H*igh-*R*isk *P*atterns of early detection (HRP). This acronym stands for heat, redness, and pain. It can develop into sepsis, a potentially fatal illness if neglected.

It's crucial to treat it right away if you suspect lymphangitis. The initial phases entail:

- **Elevate and rest the affected limb**: This can assist in relieving pain and swelling in the affected limb.
- **Use over-the-counter pain relievers** to help with pain management and fever reduction. Examples of over-the-counter pain relievers are acetaminophen and ibuprofen.

- **Sip lots of fluids**: Dehydration can increase symptoms, so drinking enough fluids can help prevent it.
- **Cleanse and bandage any open wounds**: To avoid infection, exposed wounds or sores should be cleaned and bandaged with sterile bandages.

In conclusion, addressing lymphedema consequences can be difficult, but acting quickly can help avoid major issues. Use cold packs, wipe the area, and dry it thoroughly if you suspect lymphangitis or cellulitis. Also, let your doctor know about any symptoms you experience. With the right management and care, you can lower your risk of problems and live a healthy, full life with lymphedema.

Chapter 13. The Emotional & Mental Impact of Lymphedema

My heart truly goes out to all those suffering from lymphedema. Despite the cause of your lymphedema, it's important to remember you're still in control of the outcome. Living with lymphedema is quite difficult. Let's investigate several coping mechanisms for dealing with lymphedema and its psychological effects.

As a physical therapist, I consider my patients' emotional and mental health very important. A certified lymphedema specialist will be able to guide you in all aspects of care, including where to get emotional support. In many cases, I consider myself a valuable source of emotional support.

The Effects of Lymphedema on the Psyche

Living with lymphedema can be quite emotionally taxing. It can be tricky to manage the signs and problems of lymphedema, as well as the physical changes that come along with the condition.

Among the emotional difficulties brought on by lymphedema are:

1. **Depression and anxiety**: In my years of experience, I have understood that lymphedema can trigger situational depression. So, remember your situation will improve!
2. **Social isolation**: Many patients begin isolating themselves as an unhealthy coping method. It's essential to understand this will compound your situational depression.
3. **Body image worries**: We are our own worst critics. The skin appearance and size changes, although undesirable, tend to be amplified from the perspective of the patients. The fact is most people don't notice or don't bother paying attention.
4. **Fear of recurrence**: Early stages of lymphedema, while reversible without consistent care, can return or progress into later stages. This may cause ongoing fear or worry.

Lymphedema, like any other chronic condition, can trigger the stages of grief. Denial, anger, depression, and acceptance are experienced by many lymphedema. For successful self-care at home, be aware of how lymphedema has affected you and what stage of grief you are in. In my experience, most patients tend to stay in a state of denial or depression. This becomes more evident with their behavior which may include canceling appointments, noncompliance with home exercises, and disinterest in hygiene or maintaining a clean environment. The best approach is to understand the most crucial step is the first one. Self-care at home is simple, but when you're depressed, it can seem overwhelming. So, I encourage you to engage in small steps and get involved in support groups if you notice self-sabotaging behavior.

Techniques for Managing Emotional & Mental Impact of Lymphedema

Take control of the emotional effects of lymphedema and cope with it:

1. **Seek assistance**: Assistance in managing lymphedema from family, friends, and medical professionals can be beneficial. It may be helpful to attend a support group or seek counseling. (See below)
2. **Keep moving**: Regular exercise will enhance lymphatic drainage and reduce edema. Before beginning an exercise regimen, speak with your CLT.
3. **Take good care of your skin**. Skincare can reduce the chances of infection, and a healthy appearance can boost your confidence.
4. Wear compression stockings: Many manufacturers offer a variety of styles and colors that can best suit your personality and preferences.
5. **Use relaxation methods**: Deep breathing, meditation, and yoga are all relaxation methods that can help you feel less stressed and anxious.
6. **Learn about lymphedema and how to manage it**: I am very excited you have taken the first step in taking control by purchasing this book.

Although managing lymphedema can be challenging, there are several techniques that can be useful. Stay active, take care of your skin, wear compression gear, practice relaxation techniques, and educate yourself on illness. Additionally, seek assistance from family, friends, and medical professionals. You may live a wholesome and active life despite lymphedema with the correct care and support.

Here are some support groups with thousands of members who can help:

1. Lymphedema Support Group on Facebook:
   https://www.facebook.com/groups/1043954399001286/

2. Lymphedema Support Network:
   https://www.lymphoedema.org

3. Lymphedema Treatment Act Support Group on Facebook:
   https://www.facebook.com/groups/LymphedemaTreatmentAct

Chapter 14: Living with Lymphedema

Managing lymphedema is not simple, which is why it is essential to have a solid support network. We'll examine the resources accessible to those with lymphedema in more detail in this chapter.

Support groups are one of the best options for the self-care of lymphedema at home. These clubs offer a secure and encouraging environment where members are open about their experiences and gain knowledge from others. Support groups, whether they convene in-person or online, can provide emotional support and a sense of belonging. Additionally, there are support groups created especially for families of children with lymphedema.

Organizations that support patients with lymphedema are another important source of information. These groups work to educate people about lymphedema and offer patients support, knowledge, and assistance. Several of the most well-known lymphedema patient advocacy groups include.

- The Lymphatic Research and Education Network (LE&RN)
- The National Network for Lymphedema (NLN)
- The UK-based Lymphoedema Support Network (LSN)

Lymphedema management requires the assistance of medical specialists such as physicians, physical therapists, occupational therapists, and lymphedema therapists. These experts can provide medical aid, write medication prescriptions, and offer management guidance for lymphedema. Finding qualified and experienced medical specialists who focus on treating lymphedema is crucial, though.

My company Flo-Motion serves in Orlando, Florida, and I offer virtual consultations. Please reach out to me on social media, and I can help guide you in the right direction. It would be my privilege to guide you on the path to taking control of your lymphedema. Don't hesitate.

Having access to insurance and financial resources is crucial because managing lymphedema can be financially taxing. Some lymphedema treatments, like compression garments and long-term lymphedema therapy, may not be covered by some insurance policies. For people who cannot afford lymphedema treatment, financial help options are also offered.

Here are a few examples of possible financial help programs:

- The Foundation for Patient Access Network
- The Foundation for Health and Wellness

In summary, managing lymphedema can be difficult, but there are lots of tools available to support you. Using these resources, whether support groups, patient advocacy groups, medical experts, online resources, insurance, or financial resources, can drastically improve lymphedema management. A strong support network is the secret to leading a healthy and satisfying life with lymphedema.

Chapter 15: Lymphedema Management in the Future

Lymphedema is a complicated disorder that needs constant attention to keep symptoms under control and avoid complications. Research on lymphedema has made some strides recently, as have management techniques.

Research Advances in Lymphedema

There is continuing research into the causes and treatment of lymphedema. Some current research results are as follows:

1. Surgery to reroute lymphatic vessels to promote lymphatic drainage is known as lymphatic bypass surgery. Early research points to a potential for the technique to improve lymphatic flow.
2. Using a non-invasive method called bioimpedance spectroscopy, it is possible to monitor changes in extracellular fluid. The method has been applied to track lymphedema and evaluate the treatment.
3. Exercise has been demonstrated to help ease the symptoms of lymphedema and enhance lymphatic function. According to recent studies, high-intensity interval exercise may be especially helpful for persons with lymphedema.
4. Manual lymphatic drainage (MLD) is a sort of massage that helps to increase lymphatic flow. According to recent research, compression therapy and manual lymphatic drainage are quite successful at easing the symptoms of lymphedema.

You can safely manage lymphedema at home by using YouTube as a terrific resource to learn how to implement self-massage or self-MLD into your daily life. The videos available on YouTube did not exist until recently.

Innovations in the Management of Lymphedema

In recent years there have been advancements in the treatment of lymphedema. Among these innovations are:

1. **Customized compression apparel**: Individuals' specific measurements and needs are considered when designing customized compression apparel. When it comes to lowering swelling and

increasing mobility, these garments may be superior to compression apparel available at retail stores. Almost every manufacturer offers specialized compression clothing.
2. **Pneumatic compression devices**: Pneumatic compression devices enhance lymphatic flow by applying successive pressure. These home-use tools have been proven to successfully ease the symptoms of lymphedema. Following the use of conventional decongestive therapy, most pumps are covered by insurance. Please consult your physician about acquiring a pump.
3. **Laser therapy** uses low-level laser light to enhance lymphatic flow and lessen inflammation. Early research indicates that lymphedema symptoms may be improved by laser therapy.
4. **Apps for managing lymphedema**: There are several apps for smartphones and tablets that can assist people with lymphedema. These applications can support managing compression therapy, monitoring symptoms, and gaining access to informational resources. For instance, Lymphedema Assistant or Lymphedema Self-check.
5. Researchers at the Stanford University School of Medicine may have found **a medication that can treat lymphedema**. They discovered that the medication bestatin could help alleviate lymphedema-related swelling by stimulating lymphatic vessel function. The results of this laboratory study, which used both mice and human cells, showed that bestatin was able to reduce edema significantly. Since lymphedema presently has no cure, the researchers are hopeful that this finding will spur the creation of effective new therapies. However, more research is needed to determine whether bestatin is safe and effective for treating lymphedema in individuals.

To sum up, lymphedema is a complex condition to manage, but developments in research and management techniques offer hope for those who have the condition. Recent study findings include those related to manual lymphatic drainage, exercise, bioimpedance spectroscopy, and lymphatic bypass surgery, to name just a few. Some of the most recent advancements in treating lymphedema include personalized compression clothing, pneumatic compression devices, laser therapy, and lymphedema applications. As long as research is conducted, lymphedema management will continue to develop.

Chapter 16: Final Reflections

Through a mix of self-care methods, lymphedema can be managed comfortably at home. To reduce swelling in the affected limb, the first step is to apply compression garments that may be worn all day. It's also crucial to elevate the affected limb; during the first several weeks of treatment, this should happen for 4-6 hours each day above the heart. Avoid prolonged sitting or standing with the affected limb in a dependent or down position during long-term management.

Compression and elevation are vital, but so is eating a balanced diet low in salt, processed food, and saturated fat. It's crucial to regularly moisturize and clean the skin to stop infections. The three symptoms of infection—heat, redness, and pain—should be recognized and reported to your doctor as soon as possible. Walking and active range of motion exercises for the affected leg are two exercises that can enhance circulation and lymph flow.

Remember that managing lymphedema at home needs dedication and perseverance, but it is feasible with the correct equipment and information. You may manage your lymphedema and lower the risk of problems by adhering to the five essential cornerstones of effective self-care at home. The five essentials of lymphedema self-care at home include compression, healthy diet & hydration, skincare, and exercise. Utilize the contents of this book to re-enforce the five essentials of self-care and take control of your lymphedema!

30-day Accountability Lymphedema Checklist

Name: _____   Start Date: _____

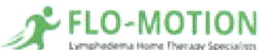

Day	Compression	Elevation	Nutrition	Exercises	Skin Care	Completed
1	[ ]	[ ]	[ ]	[ ]	[ ]	[ ]
2	[ ]	[ ]	[ ]	[ ]	[ ]	[ ]
3	[ ]	[ ]	[ ]	[ ]	[ ]	[ ]
4	[ ]	[ ]	[ ]	[ ]	[ ]	[ ]
5	[ ]	[ ]	[ ]	[ ]	[ ]	[ ]
6	[ ]	[ ]	[ ]	[ ]	[ ]	[ ]
7	[ ]	[ ]	[ ]	[ ]	[ ]	[ ]
8	[ ]	[ ]	[ ]	[ ]	[ ]	[ ]
9	[ ]	[ ]	[ ]	[ ]	[ ]	[ ]
10	[ ]	[ ]	[ ]	[ ]	[ ]	[ ]
11	[ ]	[ ]	[ ]	[ ]	[ ]	[ ]
12	[ ]	[ ]	[ ]	[ ]	[ ]	[ ]
13	[ ]	[ ]	[ ]	[ ]	[ ]	[ ]
14	[ ]	[ ]	[ ]	[ ]	[ ]	[ ]
15	[ ]	[ ]	[ ]	[ ]	[ ]	[ ]
16	[ ]	[ ]	[ ]	[ ]	[ ]	[ ]
17	[ ]	[ ]	[ ]	[ ]	[ ]	[ ]
18	[ ]	[ ]	[ ]	[ ]	[ ]	[ ]
19	[ ]	[ ]	[ ]	[ ]	[ ]	[ ]
20	[ ]	[ ]	[ ]	[ ]	[ ]	[ ]
21	[ ]	[ ]	[ ]	[ ]	[ ]	[ ]
22	[ ]	[ ]	[ ]	[ ]	[ ]	[ ]
23	[ ]	[ ]	[ ]	[ ]	[ ]	[ ]
24	[ ]	[ ]	[ ]	[ ]	[ ]	[ ]
25	[ ]	[ ]	[ ]	[ ]	[ ]	[ ]
26	[ ]	[ ]	[ ]	[ ]	[ ]	[ ]
27	[ ]	[ ]	[ ]	[ ]	[ ]	[ ]
28	[ ]	[ ]	[ ]	[ ]	[ ]	[ ]
29	[ ]	[ ]	[ ]	[ ]	[ ]	[ ]
30	[ ]	[ ]	[ ]	[ ]	[ ]	[ ]

Check off as many boxes as you can each day for 30 days. If you complete all 5 essentials of daily care, then check the completed box section for that day. Show it to your provider for review.

Resources

- https://www.ncbi.nlm.nih.gov/books/NBK537239/#:~:text=Primary%20lymphedema%20is%20rare%2C%20affecting,approximately%201%20in%201000%20Americans
- https://www.ncbi.nlm.nih.gov/pmc/articles/PMC5901432/
- https://jddonline.com/articles/a-comparison-of-physicochemical-properties-of-a-selection-of-modern-moisturizers-hydrophilic-index-a-S1545961612P0633X/#close
- National Lymphedema Network: https://lymphnet.org/
- Centers for Disease Control and Prevention: https://www.cdc.gov/
- American Society for Metabolic and Bariatric Surgery: https://asmbs.org/
- Obesity Society: https://www.obesity.org/
- Rockson SG, Granger DN, Skeff KM, Chaite W. Lymphatic biology and disease: Is it being taught? Who is listening? *Lymph at Res Biol* 2004;2:86–95
- https://www.renown.org/blog/learn-how-to-manage-lymphedema
- Women's Health Magazine: https://www.thewomenshealthmagazine.com/lymphedema-types-causes-symptoms-diagnosis-prevention-treatments-and-home-remedies/
- https://www.eatright.org/find-a-nutrition-expert
- https://www.ncbi.nlm.nih.gov/pmc/articles/PMC5787933/
- https://www.sigvaris.com/en-us/our-services/download-center/download-catalog-lookbooks
- https://www.nap.edu/read/10925/chapter/4
- https://med.stanford.edu/news/all-news/2017/05/study-finds-first-possible-drug-treatment-for-lymphedema.html#:~:text=Based%20on%20the%20research%2C%20bestatin,radiation%20therapy%2C%20trauma%20or%20infection

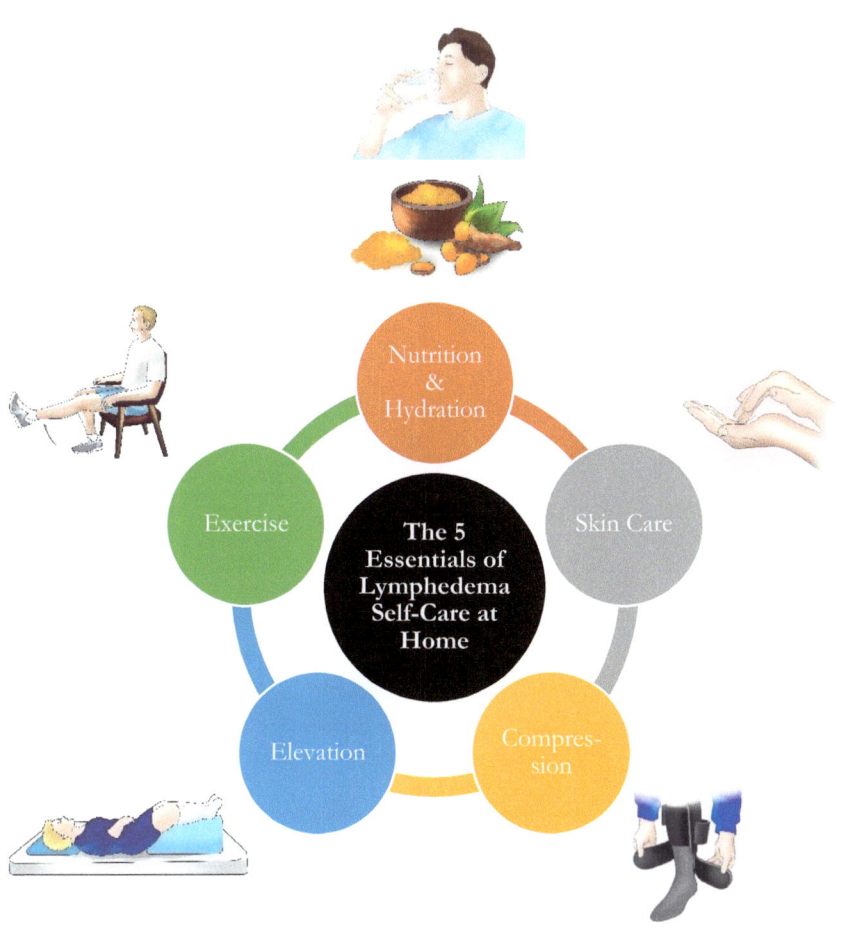

www.ingramcontent.com/pod-product-compliance
Lightning Source LLC
Chambersburg PA
CBHW040324220526
45473CB00009B/2561